GOUT DIET BOOK

Optimal Nutrition Guide to Alleviating Gout Symptoms, Reducing Inflammation, & Enhancing Your Quality of Life through Nutritious Recipes to Lower Uric Acid Levels & Reduce Flares

COURTNEY SWAN GREY

ABOUT THE AUTHOR

Hey there! I'm Courtney Swan Grey, a nutritionist with a passion for helping folks like you unlock their best health. With an M.S. in Nutrition & Integrative Health, I've been on a mission to change the way we eat and make wellness more accessible.

I believe that true health isn't just about what you eat; it's about embracing a balanced lifestyle that fuels your body, mind, and soul. Over the years, I've worked with over 500 incredible individuals, helping them lose weight, boost energy, and find their path to feeling fantastic.

My secret sauce? Tailored nutrition plans. I create plans designed just for you, understanding that your journey to wellness is unique. Plus, I'm not just a nutritionist—I'm your supportive guide and cheerleader throughout your health journey.

If you're ready to tap into your full potential for a healthier, happier life, I'm here for you. Let's embark on this exciting journey to optimal well-being together!

TABLE OF CONTENTS

INTRODUCTION

Dear Reader,

Welcome to "Gout Diet: A Comprehensive Guide to Managing Gout Through Nutrition." Whether you are someone who has recently been diagnosed with gout, a caregiver seeking information, or simply a curious individual wanting to understand this condition better, this book is your essential companion on the journey to managing gout effectively through dietary choices.

Gout, a form of arthritis, can be an incredibly painful and debilitating condition. However, with the right knowledge and lifestyle adjustments, it is a condition that can be managed, allowing you to lead a fulfilling and active life. This book has been meticulously crafted to provide you with a thorough understanding of gout and the pivotal role that diet plays in its management.

In the pages that follow, you will delve into the intricacies of gout, learning about its causes, symptoms, and complications. You will gain insights into the ways in which certain foods can trigger gout attacks and discover a wealth of information about gout-friendly foods that can help alleviate your symptoms and prevent future flare-ups.

We will guide you through the process of creating a personalized, sustainable, and enjoyable gout-friendly diet plan. From understanding portion control to exploring the benefits of superfoods and debunking common myths about gout, our aim is to empower you with the knowledge needed to make informed choices.

Moreover, this book goes beyond dietary advice. We will explore the holistic approach to managing gout, incorporating lifestyle changes, exercise routines, and stress management techniques that complement your dietary efforts. Our goal is to provide you with a comprehensive toolkit, equipping you with the skills and understanding necessary to effectively manage your gout and improve your overall quality of life.

As you embark on this educational journey, remember that you are not alone. Gaining control over your gout requires commitment, but with the right guidance, it is entirely achievable. So, let's embark on this transformative voyage together. Here's to a healthier, happier you!

CHAPTER ONE

UNDERSTANDING GOUT

What is Gout?

Gout is a form of inflammatory arthritis characterized by sudden, severe attacks of pain, redness, and tenderness in the joints, often the base of the big toe. These painful episodes, known as gout attacks, occur when urate crystals accumulate in the joints, leading to inflammation and intense discomfort.

Key Points about Gout:

Uric Acid Buildup: Gout is primarily caused by the buildup of uric acid in the bloodstream, a condition known as hyperuricemia. Uric acid is a waste product produced during the breakdown of purines, substances found in certain foods and naturally occurring in the body.

Formation of Crystals: When uric acid levels become too high, it can crystallize and deposit in joints, tendons, and surrounding tissues. These sharp urate crystals cause pain, swelling, and inflammation, leading to gout attacks.

Common Symptoms: Gout attacks often occur suddenly, usually at night, and can be triggered by factors such as alcohol consumption, certain foods, and stress. Symptoms include intense joint pain, swelling, redness, and warmth in the affected area.

Affected Joints: While the big toe is a common site for gout attacks, other joints such as ankles, knees, elbows, wrists, and fingers can also be affected. Gout can cause significant discomfort and limit mobility during an attack.

Risk Factors: Certain factors increase the risk of developing gout, including a diet rich in purine-containing foods (such as red meat and seafood), excessive alcohol consumption, obesity, high blood pressure, and a family history of gout.

Chronic Gout: If left untreated, gout can become a chronic condition, leading to frequent and prolonged gout attacks. Over time, it can cause joint damage and deformities.

Treatment and Management:

Gout can be effectively managed through lifestyle changes, dietary modifications, and, in some cases, medication. Treatment aims to reduce pain during attacks, prevent future gout attacks, and lower uric acid levels in the blood. Lifestyle changes, including a balanced diet, weight management, and regular exercise, play a crucial role in managing gout and improving overall quality of life.

Understanding the underlying causes of gout and adopting a proactive approach to its management are essential steps toward living a life with reduced pain and increased mobility.

Causes and Risk Factors

Gout, a form of arthritis, is caused by the accumulation of urate crystals in the joints, leading to inflammation and intense pain. Several factors contribute to the development of gout, and understanding these causes and risk factors is essential for effective management.

1. Uric Acid Imbalance:

Overproduction: Gout often occurs when the body produces too much uric acid, a waste product formed during the breakdown of purines found in certain foods. High levels of uric acid can lead to crystallization in the joints.

Underexcretion: In some cases, the kidneys may not efficiently excrete uric acid, causing it to build up in the bloodstream. This impaired excretion can contribute to gout development.

2. Dietary Choices:

Purine-Rich Foods: Foods high in purines, such as red meat, organ meats, seafood, and certain vegetables like spinach and asparagus, can elevate uric acid levels and trigger gout attacks.

Fructose: High intake of fructose, often found in sugary beverages, has been linked to increased uric acid levels, increasing the risk of gout.

3. Lifestyle Factors:

Alcohol Consumption: Excessive alcohol consumption, particularly beer and hard liquor, interferes with the body's ability to eliminate uric acid, making individuals more susceptible to gout.

Obesity: Being overweight increases the production of uric acid and reduces its excretion, raising the risk of developing gout.

4. Genetics and Family History:

Genetic Predisposition: Gout tends to run in families. If a close family member has gout, the risk of developing the condition is higher due to shared genetic factors.

5. Health Conditions:

Hypertension: High blood pressure is associated with an increased risk of gout. Certain medications used to treat hypertension can also raise uric acid levels.

Chronic Kidney Disease: Impaired kidney function hampers the excretion of uric acid, leading to elevated levels in the bloodstream and an increased risk of gout.

6. Age and Gender:

Age: Gout is more common in middle-aged and older adults. As people age, the risk of gout increases.

Gender: Men are more likely to develop gout, especially between the ages of 30 and 50. However, postmenopausal women also become susceptible to gout, narrowing the gender gap.

Understanding these causes and risk factors empowers individuals to make informed lifestyle choices, manage their diet effectively, and seek appropriate medical advice to prevent and manage gout successfully.

Symptoms and Diagnosis

Symptoms of Gout:

Sudden and Intense Joint Pain: Gout often manifests as a sudden, severe joint pain, most commonly in the big toe. The pain is often described as throbbing, crushing, or excruciating and can be debilitating.

Swelling and Redness: Affected joints become swollen, red, and warm to the touch. The swelling can be so pronounced that it restricts movement and causes discomfort even with the slightest touch.

Tenderness: The affected joint is extremely tender, making it painful to put any pressure on it, including the touch of clothing or sheets.

Limited Range of Motion: Due to pain and swelling, the range of motion in the affected joint is significantly reduced.

Peeling and Itching: In advanced stages or during prolonged gout attacks, the skin over the affected joint might peel and itch.

Duration and Triggers:

Gout attacks typically peak within 24 to 48 hours and can last anywhere from a few days to weeks.

Triggers for gout attacks include alcohol consumption, consuming purine-rich foods, trauma, surgery, illness, and stress.

Diagnosis of Gout:

Medical History and Physical Examination: A healthcare provider will ask about symptoms, their duration, and triggers. They will conduct a physical examination to check for swelling, redness, and tenderness in the affected joint.

Blood Tests: Blood tests measure the level of uric acid in the bloodstream. Elevated uric acid levels indicate hyperuricemia, a condition associated with gout. However, normal uric acid levels do not rule out gout, as they can fluctuate, and a gout attack can occur even with normal levels.

Joint Aspiration (Arthrocentesis): In this procedure, a small amount of fluid is extracted from the affected joint using a needle. The presence of urate crystals in the joint fluid confirms the diagnosis of gout definitively.

Imaging Studies: X-rays and ultrasound examinations can help visualize joint damage and the presence of urate crystals. These tests are particularly useful in chronic or advanced cases of gout.

Prompt and accurate diagnosis is crucial for effective management. If you experience symptoms suggestive of gout, seeking medical attention for proper evaluation and diagnosis is essential. Early diagnosis enables timely intervention, reducing the severity and frequency of gout attacks and preventing long-term joint damage.

Complications of Gout

Gout is more than just the excruciating pain of acute attacks; it can lead to various complications, some of which may have long-term consequences for your health and well-being. Understanding these complications is crucial for effective gout management.

Joint Damage: Repeated gout attacks can cause damage to the affected joints. Over time, these attacks may lead to joint deformities, limited mobility, and the development of tophi, which are lumps of urate crystals beneath the skin.

Tophi: Tophi are visible deposits of urate crystals that accumulate in the joints, tendons, and surrounding tissues. They can lead to chronic pain, joint destruction, and disfigurement.

Chronic Gout: Some individuals may develop chronic gout, characterized by frequent and prolonged gout attacks. Chronic gout can significantly impact one's quality of life and requires ongoing management.

Kidney Stones: High uric acid levels in the bloodstream can lead to the formation of urate crystals in the kidneys. These crystals may aggregate to form kidney stones, a painful condition that can result in urinary tract obstruction and infection.

Kidney Damage: In severe cases, gout can lead to kidney damage. High uric acid levels can cause inflammation and scarring in the kidneys, impairing their ability to function properly. This can result in chronic kidney disease.

Cardiovascular Complications: Gout has been associated with an increased risk of cardiovascular diseases, such as heart attacks and strokes. Chronic inflammation and high uric acid levels are believed to contribute to these risks.

Compromised Joint Function: The joint damage and chronic inflammation associated with gout can limit joint function, impacting daily activities and overall quality of life.

Psychological Impact: Gout can have a psychological impact, leading to anxiety and depression. The pain and limitations caused by gout can affect one's emotional well-being.

CHAPTER TWO

THE ROLE OF DIET IN GOUT MANAGEMENT

How Diet Affects Gout

Diet plays a pivotal role in the development and management of gout. The choices you make regarding what you eat directly influence the levels of uric acid in your bloodstream, which, in turn, can trigger or alleviate gout symptoms. Understanding how diet affects gout is essential for effectively managing this condition.

1. Purine-Rich Foods:

Effect: Purines are natural compounds found in certain foods. When you consume purine-rich foods like red meat, organ meats, seafood, and some vegetables, your body breaks down these purines into uric acid. High levels of uric acid can lead to gout attacks.

Recommendation: Limiting the intake of purine-rich foods can help reduce the risk of gout attacks. Opt for low-purine alternatives like poultry, tofu, low-fat dairy products, and vegetables like mushrooms and peas.

2. Fructose and Sugary Drinks:

Effect: Fructose, a type of sugar, increases uric acid levels in the blood. Sugary beverages, especially those high in fructose, contribute to elevated uric acid, potentially triggering gout attacks.

Recommendation: Reduce the consumption of sugary drinks, including sodas and certain fruit juices. Opt for water, herbal teas, and fresh fruit juices in moderation.

3. Alcohol:

Effect: Alcohol, particularly beer and spirits, interferes with the body's ability to excrete uric acid, leading to increased uric acid levels. Beer contains purines, making it a double risk for gout sufferers.

Recommendation: Moderation is key. If you consume alcohol, limit your intake and choose low-purine options like wine. Stay hydrated to help your body flush out uric acid.

4. Processed Foods and Saturated Fats:

Effect: Diets high in processed foods and saturated fats can contribute to obesity and insulin resistance, both of which are risk factors for gout.

Recommendation: Opt for a balanced diet rich in whole foods, fruits, vegetables, lean proteins, and whole grains. Minimize processed foods, fried foods, and foods high in saturated fats.

5. Dietary Factors that Help:

Effect: Certain foods help lower uric acid levels and reduce inflammation. These include low-fat dairy products, cherries, berries, and foods rich in vitamin C.

Recommendation: Include these gout-friendly foods in your diet. Low-fat dairy, for example, can help excrete uric acid, while cherries and berries contain compounds that may reduce inflammation and lower uric acid levels.

Foods to Avoid

1. Organ meats (liver, kidney, sweetbreads)

2. Red meat (beef, lamb, pork)

3. Game meats (venison, duck)

4. Processed meats (sausages, hot dogs)

5. Seafood (anchovies, sardines, mackerel)

6. Shellfish (shrimp, crab, lobster)

7. Gravy and meat-based sauces

8. High-purine vegetables (asparagus, spinach, mushrooms)

9. Beer

10. Spirits (whiskey, brandy)

11. Yeast extracts (yeast spreads, brewer's yeast)

12. High-fructose corn syrup (found in many sugary drinks)

13. Sugary sodas

14. Sweetened fruit juices

15. Foods high in added sugars

16. Fatty cuts of meat

17. Fried foods

18. Saturated fats (butter, lard)

19. Margarine

20. Processed snacks (chips, crisps)

21. Excessive salt

22. Caffeinated beverages (coffee, some sodas)

23. Excessive amounts of tea

24. High-fat dairy products

25. Full-fat cheese

26. High-sugar desserts (cakes, pastries)

27. Artificial sweeteners (aspartame)

28. High-purine beans (lentils)

29. Spinach

30. Cauliflower

31. Edamame

32. High-purine grains (oats, wheat bran)

33. Dried fruits (raisins, apricots)

34. High-purine condiments (soy sauce)

35. High-purine gravies

36. High-purine soups (lentil soup)

37. High-purine ready-made meals

38. Anchovy paste

39. Mussels

40. Herring

41. Lobster bisque

42. Anchovy pizza

43. Goose

44. Grilled or fried bacon

45. Mince pies

46. Beer-battered fish

47. Sweet and sour chicken

48. Chicken liver pâté

49. Pea and ham soup

50. Tuna salad sandwiches

Foods to Include

1. Low-Fat Dairy Products: (milk, yogurt, cheese)

2. Tofu

3. Eggs

4. Nuts and Seeds: (walnuts, almonds, flaxseeds, chia seeds)

5. Fruits: (cherries, strawberries, blueberries, oranges, apples)

6. Vegetables: (bell peppers, kale, cabbage, broccoli, carrots)

7. Whole Grains: (brown rice, whole wheat, quinoa, oats)

8. Legumes: (lentils, chickpeas, beans)

9. Herbs: (parsley, basil, cilantro, mint)

10. Olive Oil

11. Fatty Fish: (salmon, trout)

12. Lean Proteins: (chicken, turkey)

13. Tubers: (potatoes, sweet potatoes)

14. Avocado

15. Green Tea

16. Whole Grain Pasta

17. Mushrooms

18. Citrus Fruits: (lemons, limes, grapefruits)

19. Bananas

20. Low-Fructose Fruits: (pineapple, kiwi)

21. Celery

22. Cucumbers

23. Tomatoes

24. Onions

25. Garlic

26. Berries: (blackberries, raspberries)

27. Whole Grain Bread

28. Bell Peppers

29. Cherries

30. Low-Fat Salad Dressings

31. Herbal Teas: (chamomile, ginger)

32. Turmeric

33. Pineapple

34. Melons: (watermelon, cantaloupe)

35. Seaweed

36. Low-Fat Yogurt

37. Apricots

38. Cauliflower

39. Brussels Sprouts

40. Green Beans

41. Zucchini

42. Arugula

43. Lettuce

44. Whole Grain Cereals

45. Low-Sodium Broths

46. Unsalted Nuts

47. Low-Fat Cheese

48. Low-Fat Milk Alternatives: (almond milk, soy milk)

49. Sprouts: (alfalfa, mung bean sprouts)

50. Coconut Water

Importance of Hydration

Hydration, or maintaining adequate fluid intake, is a critical aspect of managing gout effectively. It plays a significant role in helping to prevent gout attacks and reduce the severity of symptoms. Here's why hydration is so important in gout management:

1. Uric Acid Solubility: Proper hydration helps keep uric acid in the blood more soluble. When you're well-hydrated, uric acid is less likely to crystallize and deposit in the joints, which is a major trigger for gout attacks. Hydration essentially helps to keep uric acid in solution form, reducing the risk of crystal formation.

2. Improved Uric Acid Excretion: Adequate fluid intake supports the kidneys in excreting uric acid from the body through urine. Insufficient hydration can lead to reduced uric acid excretion, allowing uric acid levels in the blood to rise, making gout attacks more likely.

3. Dilution of Toxins: Drinking plenty of water helps dilute and flush out toxins from your body, including excess uric acid. This cleansing effect reduces the concentration of uric acid in the bloodstream, making it less likely to crystallize and cause gout.

4. Prevention of Kidney Stones: Gout increases the risk of kidney stones due to the formation of urate crystals in the kidneys. Staying well-hydrated can help prevent the formation of kidney stones, which can be excruciating and detrimental to kidney health.

5. Pain and Symptom Alleviation: Proper hydration can also help alleviate the pain and inflammation associated with gout attacks. It can reduce the severity and duration of an acute gout episode.

6. General Health Benefits: Maintaining adequate hydration is essential for overall health. It supports optimal organ function, helps control body temperature, and aids in digestion and circulation.

To ensure adequate hydration for gout management, consider the following tips:

- Drink at least 8-10 cups (64-80 ounces) of water per day, or more if you're physically active or in a hot climate.
- Limit or avoid sugary, high-fructose beverages, as they can exacerbate gout.
- Include water-rich foods in your diet, such as fruits and vegetables.
- Monitor your urine color; pale yellow indicates proper hydration.

Proper hydration is a simple yet powerful tool in your arsenal for managing gout effectively. It complements dietary changes and medications, helping to reduce the frequency and intensity of gout attacks and contributing to your overall well-being.

CHAPTER THREE

CREATING A GOUT-FRIENDLY DIET PLAN

Designing a Balanced Meal Plan

Creating a balanced meal plan is crucial for effectively managing gout. A well-designed diet not only helps control uric acid levels but also provides essential nutrients and promotes overall health. Here's how to design a balanced meal plan tailored for gout management:

1. Emphasize Low-Purine Foods:

Lean Proteins: Include sources of low-purine proteins such as poultry, tofu, and eggs. These provide necessary protein without significantly raising uric acid levels.

Dairy: Opt for low-fat or fat-free dairy products. Dairy helps excrete uric acid and provides essential calcium.

Plant-Based Proteins: Legumes like lentils, chickpeas, and beans are excellent protein sources with low purine content.

2. Load Up on Vegetables and Fruits:

Colorful Variety: Include a diverse range of colorful vegetables like bell peppers, kale, and broccoli. These are rich in vitamins, minerals, and antioxidants.

Berries: Berries like cherries, strawberries, and blueberries have anti-inflammatory properties and can help lower uric acid levels.

Citrus Fruits: Oranges, lemons, and grapefruits are high in vitamin C, which may lower the risk of gout attacks.

3. Incorporate Whole Grains:

Whole Wheat: Choose whole grain options like brown rice, whole wheat bread, and whole grain pasta. These provide fiber and essential nutrients.

Quinoa: Quinoa is a complete protein and a good alternative to purine-rich grains.

4. Healthy Fats:

Olive Oil: Use olive oil for cooking and in dressings. It contains monounsaturated fats, which are heart-healthy.

Nuts and Seeds: Include almonds, walnuts, and flaxseeds for healthy fats and omega-3 fatty acids.

5. Limit Purine-Rich Foods:

Red Meat: Minimize intake of red meats like beef, lamb, and pork.

Seafood: Avoid high-purine seafood such as anchovies, sardines, and mackerel.

Organ Meats: Completely avoid organ meats like liver and kidney.

6. Stay Hydrated:

Water: Drink plenty of water throughout the day. Proper hydration helps in flushing out uric acid from the body.

7. Portion Control and Moderation:

Balanced Portions: Pay attention to portion sizes to maintain a healthy weight. Avoid overeating, especially high-calorie foods.

Moderate Alcohol: If you choose to drink alcohol, do so in moderation. Limit beer and spirits, opting for wine in small amounts if desired.

8. Meal Timing:

Regular Meals: Aim for regular meal times to maintain stable energy levels and prevent overeating.

Avoid Fasting: Prolonged fasting or crash diets can increase uric acid levels.

Weekly Meal Prep Tips

Preparing your meals in advance not only saves time but also ensures that you have healthy, gout-friendly options readily available. Here are some helpful tips for successful weekly meal prep tailored for managing gout:

1. Plan Your Meals:

Create a Menu: Plan your meals for the week, including breakfast, lunch, dinner, and snacks. Consider recipes that incorporate low-purine foods and a variety of vegetables and fruits.

Balance Your Nutrients: Ensure your meals include a balance of lean proteins, whole grains, vegetables, and healthy fats. This balance is essential for managing gout effectively.

2. Batch Cooking:

Prepare Proteins: Cook a batch of lean proteins like chicken, tofu, or beans. Divide them into portions for various meals throughout the week.

Cook Whole Grains: Cook a large batch of whole grains such as brown rice or quinoa. These can serve as a base for multiple dishes.

Chop Vegetables: Wash, peel, and chop vegetables like bell peppers, carrots, and broccoli. Store them in containers for quick use in salads, stir-fries, or snacks.

3. Prep Gout-Friendly Snacks:

Portion Nuts and Seeds: Divide nuts and seeds like almonds and walnuts into small portions for snacking. These are healthy sources of fats and protein.

Prepare Fresh Fruit: Wash and cut fruits like berries, melons, and citrus fruits. Having them readily available encourages healthy snacking.

4. Prepare Gout-Friendly Sauces and Dressings:

Homemade Sauces: Prepare low-fat and low-sodium sauces using fresh herbs, tomatoes, and olive oil. Avoid high-purine sauces.

Healthy Dressings: Make vinaigrettes using olive oil, lemon juice, and herbs. Avoid commercial dressings high in sugars and unhealthy fats.

5. Use Portion-Controlled Containers:

Invest in Containers: Use portion-controlled containers to store your meals. This prevents overeating and helps maintain balanced portions.

Label and Date: Label the containers with the meal content and date of preparation to keep track of freshness.

6. Include Gout-Friendly Beverages:

Infused Water: Infuse water with fruits like lemon, lime, or cucumber for added flavor without added sugars.

Herbal Teas: Prepare herbal teas like chamomile or ginger, which are hydrating and have potential anti-inflammatory properties.

7. Avoid Excessive Salt and Sugar:

Read Labels: When using packaged ingredients, check labels for hidden salts and sugars. Excessive salt and sugar intake can exacerbate gout symptoms.

Opt for Fresh: Whenever possible, use fresh ingredients. Fresh produce, lean meats, and whole grains are naturally low in salt and sugar.

8. Stay Organized:

Meal Prep Schedule: Dedicate a specific day and time each week for meal prep. Consistency helps in creating a routine.

Inventory Check: Before grocery shopping, check your pantry and fridge. Knowing what you have reduces waste and ensures you use existing ingredients.

9. Experiment with Recipes:

Explore New Recipes: Experiment with gout-friendly recipes to keep your meals interesting. There are numerous creative and healthy recipes available online.

Plan Variety: Include a variety of cuisines and flavors in your meal plan to prevent culinary monotony.

10. Stay Flexible:

Adapt to Your Needs: Be flexible with your meal plan. If you have leftovers, incorporate them into the next day's meal. Adapt recipes to suit your taste and dietary preferences.

Portion Control and Calorie Management

Proper portion control and calorie management are essential components of a gout-friendly diet. Balancing your intake helps maintain a healthy weight and can reduce the risk of gout attacks. Here's how to approach portion control and calorie management effectively:

1. Understand Serving Sizes:

Read Labels: Pay attention to serving sizes on food labels. They provide guidelines for portion control and help you understand the calorie content per serving.

Use Measuring Tools: Invest in measuring cups and a kitchen scale. Measuring ingredients ensures accuracy and prevents overeating.

2. Mindful Eating:

Eat Slowly: Chew your food slowly and savor each bite. Eating too quickly may lead to overeating.

Listen to Your Body: Pay attention to your body's hunger and fullness cues. Stop eating when you feel satisfied, not overly full.

3. Balanced Plate Approach:

Visualize Your Plate: Aim to fill half your plate with vegetables and fruits, one-quarter with lean proteins, and one-quarter with whole grains.

Avoid Oversized Plates: Use smaller plates to create the illusion of a fuller plate, which can help control portion sizes.

4. Caloric Intake:

Calculate Your Needs: Determine your daily caloric needs based on factors like age, gender, activity level, and weight goals.

Create a Calorie Deficit: If weight loss is a goal, create a calorie deficit by consuming fewer calories than you burn through physical activity and daily functions.

5. Avoid Empty Calories:

Limit Sugary Foods: Reduce intake of sugary beverages, candies, and desserts. These provide empty calories and can contribute to weight gain.

Limit Processed Foods: Processed foods often contain high levels of added sugars and unhealthy fats. Opt for whole, unprocessed foods.

6. Healthy Snacking:

Plan Snacks: If snacking is part of your routine, plan healthy snacks like fresh fruits, nuts, or yogurt. Portion them out in advance to avoid mindless eating.

Hydration: Sometimes, feelings of hunger are actually signs of dehydration. Stay hydrated with water or herbal teas to manage unnecessary snacking.

7. Avoid Emotional Eating:

Identify Triggers: Be aware of emotional triggers that lead to overeating. Find alternative ways to cope with stress, boredom, or sadness that don't involve food.

Practice Mindfulness: Engage in mindfulness practices, such as meditation or yoga, to develop a healthier relationship with food.

CHAPTER FOUR

GOUT-TRIGGERING FOODS: WHAT TO AVOID

High-Purine Foods and Gout

1. Organ Meats:

Examples: Liver, kidney, and sweetbreads. These are exceptionally high in purines and should be avoided or consumed in very limited quantities.

2. Red Meats:

Examples: Beef, lamb, and pork. While these are protein-rich, they are also high in purines. Moderation is key.

3. Seafood:

High-Purine Varieties: Anchovies, sardines, mackerel, herring, trout, and scallops. These types of seafood have high purine content and can lead to elevated uric acid levels.

4. Shellfish:

Examples: Shrimp, crab, lobster, and clams. While shellfish are a popular choice, they are also purine-rich and should be limited.

5. Game Meats:

Examples: Venison, duck, and goose. These meats, often considered delicacies, are high in purines and should be consumed sparingly.

6. Yeast Extracts:

Examples: Yeast spreads, extracts, and supplements. These products, often used in cooking, can contribute to elevated uric acid levels.

7. Certain Vegetables:

High-Purine Vegetables: Asparagus, spinach, cauliflower, and mushrooms. While vegetables are generally healthy, these specific ones have moderate to high purine content.

8. Alcohol:

Beer: Beer, particularly craft beers, is associated with a higher risk of gout due to its purine content and its influence on uric acid metabolism.

Spirits: Some studies suggest that spirits, especially when consumed in excess, can increase the likelihood of gout attacks.

9. Fructose:

High-Fructose Corn Syrup (HFCS): Found in many processed foods and sugary beverages, HFCS can lead to elevated uric acid levels, increasing the risk of gout attacks.

For individuals with gout, it's crucial to limit these high-purine foods and beverages. A balanced diet that focuses on low-purine alternatives, including lean proteins, whole grains, fruits, vegetables, and low-fat dairy products, can help manage uric acid levels effectively. Additionally, staying well-hydrated and maintaining a healthy weight are integral parts of gout management, providing a comprehensive approach to minimizing gout attacks and maintaining joint health.

Red Meat and Gout Attacks

Red meat, including beef, lamb, and pork, is rich in purines, natural compounds that break down into uric acid. High levels of uric acid can lead to the formation of urate crystals in the joints, triggering gout attacks. Here's how red meat contributes to gout:

1. High Purine Content:

Purines in Red Meat: Red meat is one of the highest purine-containing foods. When you consume red meat, your body breaks down these purines, leading to an increase in uric acid levels in the bloodstream.

Uric Acid Buildup: Elevated uric acid levels can result in the formation of urate crystals, which can accumulate in the joints, causing pain, swelling, and inflammation characteristic of gout attacks.

2. Effects on Uric Acid Metabolism:

Red Meat and Uric Acid Production: Red meat consumption not only introduces purines into the body but also affects uric acid metabolism. Some components in red meat can hinder the kidneys' ability to excrete uric acid efficiently.

3. Increased Risk with Overconsumption:

Portion Sizes and Frequency: Larger portions of red meat and frequent consumption can significantly raise uric acid levels. Overindulgence, especially in fatty cuts, intensifies the risk of gout attacks.

Managing Red Meat Consumption:

For individuals prone to gout attacks or those diagnosed with gout, managing red meat intake is vital:

1. Limit Portion Sizes:

Moderation is Key: If you choose to consume red meat, do so in small, controlled portions. Avoid excessive servings that can overload your system with purines.

2. Choose Lean Cuts:

Lean Proteins: Opt for lean cuts of red meat, trimming visible fat. Lean meats contain fewer purines and are healthier choices for individuals with gout.

3. Balance with Plant-Based Proteins:

Alternative Proteins: Incorporate plant-based proteins like legumes, tofu, and tempeh into your diet. These options are lower in purines and provide excellent alternatives to red meat.

Seafood and Gout Flare-Ups

Seafood is a broad category that includes a variety of fish and shellfish. Some types of seafood have high purine content, leading to elevated uric acid levels and potentially causing gout attacks. Here's what you need to know:

1. High-Purine Seafood:

Examples: Anchovies, sardines, mackerel, herring, trout, and scallops. These types of fish and shellfish are rich in purines and can contribute to gout flare-ups when consumed in excess.

2. Moderate-Purine Seafood:

Examples: Salmon, tuna, and shrimp. While these are lower in purines compared to high-purine seafood, moderation is still essential, especially for individuals prone to gout attacks.

3. Purine Breakdown:

Purines to Uric Acid: When you consume seafood high in purines, your body breaks down these purines into uric acid. Elevated uric acid levels can lead to the formation of urate crystals, triggering gout symptoms.

Managing Seafood Consumption:

For individuals with gout or those at risk, being mindful of seafood choices can help prevent gout flare-ups:

1. Limit High-Purine Seafood:

Avoidance or Moderation: Limit or avoid high-purine seafood like anchovies, mackerel, and sardines. If you choose to consume them, do so in small quantities and infrequently.

2. Choose Lower-Purine Alternatives:

Safe Choices: Opt for lower-purine seafood such as salmon, tuna, and shrimp. These options are safer for individuals with gout when consumed in moderation.

3. Balanced Diet:

Variety is Key: Include a variety of protein sources in your diet. Balance seafood consumption with lean meats, poultry, tofu, legumes, and dairy for a diverse and balanced protein intake.

Alcohol, Sugary Drinks, and Gout

Alcohol consumption, especially beer and spirits, can significantly increase the risk of gout attacks for several reasons:

1. **Purine Content:** Some alcoholic beverages, particularly beer, contain high levels of purines, which

metabolize into uric acid. This can lead to elevated uric acid levels and gout attacks.

2. Decreased Uric Acid Excretion: Alcohol can impair the kidneys' ability to excrete uric acid efficiently, leading to its accumulation in the bloodstream.

3. Dehydration: Alcohol is a diuretic, meaning it increases urine production and can lead to dehydration. Dehydration can concentrate uric acid in the body, increasing the risk of gout flare-ups.

4. Increased Risk with Overindulgence: Excessive alcohol consumption, even of low-purine beverages, can overload the body's ability to process uric acid, heightening the risk of gout attacks.

Sugary Drinks and Gout:

Sugary beverages, including sodas and certain fruit juices, are associated with a higher risk of gout attacks due to several factors:

1. Fructose Content: Fructose, a type of sugar found in high-fructose corn syrup (HFCS), increases uric acid levels in the blood. Beverages sweetened with HFCS can lead to elevated uric acid and gout attacks.

2. Insulin Resistance: High consumption of sugary drinks can contribute to insulin resistance and obesity, both of which are risk factors for gout.

3. Empty Calories: Sugary drinks are high in calories but lack essential nutrients. Excessive consumption can lead to weight gain and exacerbate gout symptoms.

Managing Alcohol and Sugary Drink Intake:

For individuals with gout or those at risk, it's crucial to approach alcohol and sugary beverages mindfully:

1. Moderation is Key:

Limit Alcohol: If you choose to drink, do so in moderation. Limit beer and spirits, opting for wine in small amounts if desired.

Reduce Sugary Drinks: Cut back on sodas, sweetened teas, and fruit juices. Opt for water, herbal teas, or beverages sweetened with natural, low-calorie sweeteners.

2. Stay Hydrated:

Water Intake: Drink plenty of water throughout the day. Proper hydration helps flush out uric acid and reduce the risk of gout attacks.

3. **Read Labels:**

Check Sugar Content: When buying beverages, read labels to identify added sugars and choose low-sugar or sugar-free options.

CHAPTER FIVE

INCORPORATING SUPERFOODS INTO YOUR GOUT DIET

Berries and Their Anti-Inflammatory Properties

Berries, including strawberries, blueberries, raspberries, and blackberries, are not only delicious but also packed with essential nutrients and antioxidants. One of the key health benefits associated with berries is their remarkable anti-inflammatory properties. Here's how these tiny fruits can play a significant role in promoting overall well-being:

1. Rich in Antioxidants:

Anthocyanins: Berries, especially blueberries, owe their vibrant colors to compounds called anthocyanins, which possess potent antioxidant and anti-inflammatory effects. These antioxidants help neutralize harmful free radicals in the body, reducing oxidative stress and inflammation.

2. Anti-Inflammatory Compounds:

Flavonoids: Berries are rich in flavonoids, a group of bioactive compounds known for their anti-inflammatory properties. These flavonoids inhibit certain enzymes that promote inflammation, helping to mitigate chronic inflammation in the body.

3. Reduced Risk of Chronic Diseases:

Cardiovascular Health: Regular consumption of berries has been linked to improved heart health. The antioxidants in berries help lower blood pressure, reduce cholesterol levels, and prevent the oxidation of LDL cholesterol, all of which contribute to a reduced risk of cardiovascular diseases.

Brain Health: Anthocyanins found in berries have been associated with a lower risk of age-related cognitive decline. They may improve memory and cognitive function by protecting brain cells from inflammation and oxidative stress.

Cancer Prevention: Some studies suggest that the compounds in berries may have protective effects against certain types of cancer due to their anti-inflammatory and antioxidant properties.

4. Fighting Joint Inflammation:

Arthritis Management: The anti-inflammatory effects of berries can be particularly beneficial for individuals with arthritis. Regular consumption may help reduce joint pain and inflammation associated with arthritis, improving overall joint health and mobility.

5. Including Berries in Your Diet:

Fresh or Frozen: Berries are widely available fresh or frozen, making it convenient to incorporate them into your diet year-round.

Smoothies: Add a handful of berries to your morning smoothies for a burst of antioxidants and natural sweetness.

Yogurt and Oatmeal: Top your yogurt or oatmeal with mixed berries for a nutritious and flavorful addition.

Salads: Berries can add a refreshing twist to salads, pairing well with greens, nuts, and cheese.

Snacking: Enjoy berries as a healthy snack on their own or mixed with other fruits and nuts.

By including a variety of berries in your diet, you can harness their anti-inflammatory properties, promoting overall health and potentially reducing the risk of chronic diseases. Whether enjoyed on their own or incorporated into recipes, these nutrient-packed fruits offer a delicious way to support your well-being.

Leafy Greens and Gout Prevention

Leafy greens, such as spinach, kale, lettuce, and Swiss chard, are nutritional powerhouses that offer numerous health benefits, including their potential role in gout prevention. Here's how these vibrant vegetables can contribute to joint health and assist in managing gout:

1. Low in Purines:

Gout-Friendly Choice: Leafy greens are naturally low in purines, the compounds that break down into uric acid and can trigger gout attacks. Including these greens in your diet helps maintain lower uric acid levels, reducing the risk of gout flare-ups.

2. Rich in Vitamin C:

Anti-Gout Properties: Leafy greens, particularly spinach and kale, are excellent sources of vitamin C. Vitamin C has been shown to lower uric acid levels in the blood, making it beneficial for individuals with gout. Adequate intake of vitamin C can help prevent uric acid crystal formation in the joints.

3. High in Fiber:

Digestive Health: Leafy greens are high in dietary fiber, promoting healthy digestion and regular bowel movements. Adequate fiber intake assists in the elimination of waste products, including uric acid, from the body.

4. Rich in Anti-Inflammatory Compounds:

Phytonutrients: Leafy greens contain various phytonutrients, such as flavonoids and carotenoids, with anti-inflammatory properties. These compounds help reduce inflammation in the body, including joint inflammation associated with gout.

5. Weight Management:

Low-Calorie, Nutrient-Dense: Leafy greens are low in calories but high in essential vitamins and minerals. Including them in your diet supports weight management, as they provide vital nutrients without adding excess calories. Maintaining a healthy weight is crucial for gout prevention, as obesity is a risk factor for the condition.

6. Versatile and Delicious:

Creative Cooking: Leafy greens can be incorporated into a variety of dishes, including salads, soups, smoothies, and stir-fries. Experimenting with different cooking methods keeps your meals exciting and ensures a consistent intake of these nutritious greens.

7. Balanced Diet Approach:

Dietary Diversity: In combination with other gout-friendly foods, such as low-fat dairy products, whole grains, and fruits, leafy greens contribute to a well-balanced, nutritious diet. A diverse diet supports overall health and gout prevention.

Nuts, Seeds, and Omega-3 Fatty Acids

Nuts and seeds are not only delicious snacks but also valuable sources of essential nutrients, including omega-3 fatty acids. Incorporating these nutrient-rich foods into your diet can have significant benefits for joint health and overall well-being, especially for individuals managing conditions like gout. Here's why nuts, seeds, and omega-3 fatty acids are nutritional allies for joint health:

1. Omega-3 Fatty Acids:

Anti-Inflammatory Properties: Nuts and seeds, particularly flaxseeds, chia seeds, and walnuts, are rich in alpha-linolenic acid (ALA), a type of omega-3 fatty acid. Omega-3s have potent anti-inflammatory effects, reducing joint inflammation and potentially alleviating symptoms associated with gout and other inflammatory conditions.

Joint Lubrication: Omega-3s contribute to joint lubrication and flexibility. Adequate intake can improve joint function and reduce stiffness, enhancing overall joint mobility.

2. Nuts and Seeds:

Healthy Fats: Nuts, such as almonds, pistachios, and hazelnuts, and seeds like flaxseeds, chia seeds, and pumpkin seeds, are excellent sources of healthy monounsaturated and polyunsaturated fats. These fats are heart-healthy and can help reduce inflammation in the body, including in the joints.

Protein and Fiber: Nuts and seeds are also good sources of plant-based proteins and dietary fiber. Protein is essential for muscle and tissue repair, while fiber aids in digestion and the elimination of waste products, promoting overall gut health.

3. Incorporating Nuts and Seeds:

Snacking: Enjoy a handful of mixed nuts or seeds as a snack between meals. They provide sustained energy and are convenient to carry.

Smoothies: Add a tablespoon of ground flaxseeds or chia seeds to your smoothies for a boost of omega-3s and a pleasant texture.

Salads: Sprinkle chopped nuts or seeds over salads for added crunch and a nutrient boost.

Baking: Incorporate nuts and seeds into baking recipes, such as whole grain muffins or homemade granola bars, for extra flavor and nutrition.

4. Supplementation:

Consideration: If it's challenging to obtain omega-3s from food sources, consider omega-3 supplements after consulting with a healthcare provider. However, getting nutrients from whole foods is generally recommended for optimal absorption and health benefits.

Herbal Teas and Gout Relief

Herbal teas have long been cherished for their therapeutic properties, and when it comes to gout relief, certain herbal teas can be particularly beneficial. While herbal teas are not a substitute for medical treatment, they can play a supportive role in managing gout symptoms. Here are some herbal teas known for their potential in providing gout relief:

1. Chamomile Tea:

Anti-Inflammatory: Chamomile tea is renowned for its anti-inflammatory properties. It can help reduce joint inflammation and provide relief from gout-related pain and discomfort. Its calming effects also promote relaxation, which is beneficial during gout attacks.

2. Ginger Tea:

Pain Relief: Ginger tea possesses natural anti-inflammatory and analgesic (pain-relieving) properties. It can help alleviate joint pain associated with gout and promote overall joint health. Ginger's warming effect can also enhance blood circulation.

3. Turmeric Tea:

Curcumin Content: Turmeric contains curcumin, a potent anti-inflammatory compound. Turmeric tea can help reduce inflammation, making it useful for managing gout symptoms. Its antioxidant properties also contribute to overall joint health.

4. Nettle Leaf Tea:

Natural Diuretic: Nettle leaf tea acts as a natural diuretic, promoting the elimination of excess uric acid and waste products from the body. By supporting kidney function, nettle leaf tea can potentially reduce the risk of gout attacks.

5. Celery Seed Tea:

Anti-Gout Properties: Celery seeds have been traditionally used for gout relief due to their diuretic properties and potential to lower uric acid levels. Brewing celery seed tea can be an effective way to incorporate this natural remedy into your routine.

6. Burdock Root Tea:

Detoxification: Burdock root tea is believed to support detoxification by aiding the liver and kidneys in removing toxins and excess uric acid from the body. By promoting cleansing, it may contribute to gout symptom relief.

7. Dandelion Tea:

Diuretic Effect: Dandelion tea acts as a gentle diuretic, promoting increased urination. This can help flush out uric acid and reduce water retention, potentially providing relief from gout symptoms.

CHAPTER SIX

LIFESTYLE CHANGES FOR GOUT MANAGEMENT

Exercise and Gout Prevention

1. Low-Impact Aerobic Exercises:

Walking: A brisk walk is a low-impact exercise that improves cardiovascular health and joint mobility without putting excessive stress on the joints.

Swimming: Swimming and water aerobics provide a full-body workout while being gentle on the joints. The buoyancy of water reduces impact and supports joint movement.

Cycling: Riding a stationary bike or cycling outdoors offers an effective cardiovascular workout while being easy on the joints.

2. Strength Training:

Bodyweight Exercises: Bodyweight exercises like squats, lunges, push-ups, and planks help build muscle strength and improve overall stability.

Resistance Bands: Resistance band exercises target specific muscle groups, aiding in strength development without putting excessive strain on the joints.

Light Weights: Using light dumbbells or resistance machines can help increase muscle strength. Focus on proper form and controlled movements.

3. Flexibility and Range of Motion Exercises:

Yoga: Yoga poses enhance flexibility, balance, and joint mobility. It also promotes relaxation and stress reduction.

Tai Chi: Tai Chi combines gentle movements and deep breathing, enhancing balance, flexibility, and overall body awareness.

Stretching: Regular stretching exercises improve joint flexibility and reduce muscle tension. Include dynamic and static stretches in your routine.

4. Balance and Coordination Exercises:

Balance Exercises: Activities like standing on one leg, using balance boards, or stability ball exercises enhance balance and stability, reducing the risk of falls.

Coordination Drills: Engage in activities that challenge hand-eye coordination, such as catching and throwing a ball or playing table tennis.

5. Adequate Warm-Up and Cool-Down:

Warm-Up: Always start your exercise session with a gentle warm-up to prepare your muscles and joints. This can include light aerobic activity and dynamic stretching.

Cool Down: Finish your workout with a cool-down period, incorporating static stretching to improve flexibility and prevent muscle soreness.

6. Regular Physical Activity Recommendations:

Frequency: Aim for at least 150 minutes of moderate-intensity aerobic exercise per week, spread across several days.

Consistency: Consistency is key. Engage in regular physical activity to maintain joint health and overall well-being.

Consultation: Before starting a new exercise program, especially if you have underlying health conditions, consult a healthcare provider or a certified fitness professional for personalized recommendations.

Stress Management Techniques

In today's fast-paced world, effective stress management techniques are essential for maintaining mental, emotional, and physical well-being. Here are various techniques that can help you manage stress and promote a sense of calm and balance in your life:

1. Mindfulness Meditation:

Focused Breathing: Practice mindful breathing exercises, focusing on your breath to bring your attention to the present moment. Inhale deeply and exhale slowly, allowing yourself to relax with each breath.

Body Scan: Conduct a mental scan of your body, paying attention to areas of tension. Breathe into these areas, allowing the tension to dissolve as you exhale.

Guided Meditation: Listen to guided meditation sessions that help you relax and cultivate mindfulness. Many apps and online platforms offer guided meditation recordings.

2. Yoga and Tai Chi:

Yoga: Yoga combines physical postures, breathing exercises, and meditation, promoting flexibility, strength, and relaxation.

Tai Chi: Tai Chi is a gentle form of martial arts that involves slow, flowing movements and deep breathing. It enhances balance, flexibility, and inner peace.

3. Physical Activity:

Regular Exercise: Engage in regular physical activity, such as walking, jogging, swimming, or dancing. Exercise releases endorphins, which are natural stress relievers.

Dance and Music: Dancing to your favorite music can be a joyful and expressive way to release stress and boost your mood.

4. Art and Creativity:

Drawing and Painting: Engage in art activities, even if you're not an artist. Drawing and painting can serve as creative outlets, allowing you to express emotions and thoughts.

Crafting: Try knitting, crocheting, or other crafting activities. Engaging in repetitive, creative tasks can be meditative and soothing.

5. Connecting with Nature:

Nature Walks: Spend time in nature. Take leisurely walks in parks or natural surroundings, appreciating the beauty of the outdoors.

Gardening: Gardening can be therapeutic. Tending to plants and flowers allows you to connect with the earth and experience a sense of fulfillment.

6. Social Support:

Talk to Loved Ones: Reach out to friends, family, or a supportive community. Sharing your feelings with others can provide comfort and perspective.

Support Groups: Consider joining a support group, either in person or online, where you can connect with others facing similar challenges.

7. Relaxation Techniques:

Deep Breathing: Practice deep breathing exercises to calm your mind and body. Inhale slowly, hold your breath briefly, and then exhale slowly, releasing tension with each breath.

Progressive Muscle Relaxation: Tense and then relax different muscle groups in your body, starting from your toes and moving upward. This technique helps release physical tension.

8. Mindfulness Practices:

Mindful Eating: Practice mindful eating by savoring each bite, paying attention to taste, texture, and aroma. Eating mindfully can enhance your relationship with food and reduce stress-related overeating.

Gratitude Journaling: Keep a gratitude journal, noting down things you are thankful for each day. Focusing on positive aspects of your life can shift your perspective and reduce stress.

9. Setting Boundaries:

Learn to Say No: Set realistic limits on what you can and cannot do. Learn to say no to additional commitments that may overwhelm you.

Prioritize Self-Care: Make time for self-care activities that bring you joy and relaxation, whether it's reading, taking a bath, or spending time with hobbies.

Getting Adequate Sleep

Quality sleep is essential for overall health and well-being. It plays a crucial role in physical, mental, and emotional functioning. Here are key practices to ensure you get the restful sleep your body and mind need:

1. Establish a Sleep Schedule:

Consistent Bedtime: Go to bed and wake up at the same time every day, even on weekends. Consistency helps regulate your body's internal clock, enhancing the quality of your sleep.

Create a Bedtime Ritual: Engage in relaxing activities before bedtime, such as reading, taking a warm bath, or practicing gentle yoga. Establishing a calming routine signals to your body that it's time to wind down.

2. Create a Sleep-Friendly Environment:

Comfortable Mattress and Pillow: Invest in a comfortable mattress and supportive pillows that suit your sleep preferences. A good mattress supports your spine's natural alignment.

Dark and Quiet: Make your bedroom conducive to sleep by keeping it dark, quiet, and cool. Consider using blackout curtains and white noise machines if needed.

Limit Electronic Devices: Reduce exposure to screens (phones, tablets, computers) at least an hour before bedtime. The blue light emitted by electronic devices can interfere with your sleep-wake cycle.

3. Watch Your Diet and Hydration:

Limit Caffeine and Alcohol: Avoid caffeine and alcohol in the hours leading up to bedtime. Both can disrupt your sleep cycle and affect the quality of your rest.

Avoid Heavy Meals: Large or spicy meals close to bedtime can cause discomfort and indigestion, making it harder to fall asleep. Opt for a light snack if you're hungry.

4. Regular Exercise:

Morning Exercise: Engage in physical activity regularly, but aim to complete your workouts earlier in the day. Exercise helps regulate your sleep patterns and promotes a deeper, more restorative sleep.

5. Manage Stress:

Relaxation Techniques: Practice relaxation methods such as deep breathing, meditation, or gentle stretching before bedtime. These techniques can help calm your mind and prepare your body for sleep.

Journaling: Consider jotting down your thoughts or worries in a journal before bedtime. This practice can help clear your mind and reduce anxiety.

6. Limit Naps:

Daytime Naps: If you need to nap during the day, limit it to a short duration (20-30 minutes) and avoid napping late in the afternoon, as it can interfere with your ability to fall asleep at night.

Importance of Regular Medical Checkups

Regular medical checkups are fundamental to maintaining good health and preventing potential health issues. Here's why scheduling routine appointments with healthcare providers is crucial:

1. Early Detection of Health Conditions:

Preventive Screenings: Regular checkups often include screenings for conditions like high blood pressure, cholesterol levels, diabetes, and certain cancers. Early detection allows for timely intervention and better management of these conditions.

2. Preventive Care and Immunizations:

Vaccinations: Healthcare providers can ensure you're up-to-date with necessary vaccinations, protecting you from various diseases and promoting community immunity.

Preventive Counseling: Doctors provide guidance on healthy lifestyle choices, nutrition, exercise, and stress management, empowering you to make informed decisions about your well-being.

3. Management of Chronic Conditions:

Chronic Disease Management: For individuals with chronic conditions like diabetes, hypertension, or arthritis, regular checkups help monitor the condition's progression, adjust medications, and provide necessary support and guidance.

Medication Management: Healthcare providers can review your medications, assess their effectiveness, and address any side effects, ensuring you're on the right treatment plan.

4. Mental Health Support:

Mental Health Checkups: Mental health is as vital as physical health. Healthcare providers can assess your mental well-being, offer support, and connect you with mental health professionals if needed.

Counseling and Therapy: Regular checkups provide an opportunity to discuss stress, anxiety, or depression. Healthcare providers can recommend therapy or counseling services as appropriate.

5. Continuity of Care:

Comprehensive Health Records: Regular medical visits contribute to a comprehensive medical history. This information is invaluable in emergencies, ensuring healthcare providers have a complete understanding of your health profile.

Effective Communication: Establishing a rapport with your healthcare provider fosters open communication. You can freely discuss concerns, symptoms, or lifestyle changes, enabling better diagnosis and personalized care.

6. Health Education and Awareness:

Health Literacy: Medical professionals educate patients about their health conditions, treatments, and preventive measures. Understanding your health empowers you to actively participate in your care.

Awareness of Risk Factors: Doctors can assess your risk factors based on family history, lifestyle, and overall health, guiding you in making lifestyle changes to minimize these risks.

7. Timely Referrals and Specialized Care:

Specialist Referrals: If necessary, healthcare providers can refer you to specialists for specific evaluations or treatments, ensuring you receive specialized care when needed.

Coordination of Care: Regular checkups facilitate coordination between healthcare providers, ensuring seamless care, especially if you have multiple health conditions.

8. Quality of Life and Longevity:

Healthy Aging: Regular medical checkups contribute to healthy aging by addressing age-related concerns, and monitoring bone health, vision, and cognitive function.

Enhanced Quality of Life: By addressing health issues promptly, regular checkups enhance your quality of life, allowing you to enjoy daily activities and pursue your passions.

CHAPTER SEVEN

GOUT DIET FOR DIFFERENT LIFESTAGES

Gout in Young Adults

Surprising Onset: While gout is often associated with older adults, it can also affect young adults, particularly those with a family history of the condition or individuals leading unhealthy lifestyles.

Contributing Factors: Factors like excessive alcohol consumption, high intake of purine-rich foods, obesity, and certain genetic predispositions can lead to gout in young adults.

Impact on Lifestyle: Gout in young adults can significantly impact daily activities and may require lifestyle modifications, medication, and dietary changes to manage symptoms and prevent future attacks.

Gout in Middle-Aged Individuals

Peak Occurrence: Gout is most commonly diagnosed in middle-aged individuals, often between the ages of 30 and 60.

Lifestyle Factors: Poor dietary choices, sedentary lifestyles, obesity, and hypertension often contribute to gout in middle age.

Management and Prevention: Middle-aged individuals with gout benefit from a combination of medication, dietary adjustments (low-purine diet), weight management, and regular exercise to manage symptoms and prevent recurrent attacks.

Gout in Seniors

Increased Prevalence: Gout becomes more prevalent as people age, partly due to changes in metabolism and the body's ability to excrete uric acid effectively.

Comorbidity Challenges: Seniors with gout often have other health conditions, complicating the management of gout. Medication management should consider these factors to avoid adverse drug interactions.

Joint Damage Concerns: Long-term gout can lead to joint damage and deformities in seniors. Early diagnosis, lifestyle modifications, and adherence to prescribed medications are crucial for preventing complications.

. Gout and Women: Special Considerations

Hormonal Influence: Gout is less common in women compared to men, but hormonal changes (such as menopause) can increase uric acid levels, raising the risk of gout attacks.

Pregnancy and Gout: Gout management during pregnancy requires careful consideration due to restrictions on certain medications. Lifestyle modifications and dietary changes become primary methods of management.

Impact on Quality of Life: Gout can affect women's quality of life significantly. Women may face unique challenges related to family planning, lifestyle adjustments, and psychological well-being when managing gout.

Key Takeaways:

- **Early Intervention:** Regardless of age or gender, early diagnosis and management of gout are essential to prevent joint damage and enhance overall quality of life.

- **Holistic Approach:** Gout management involves a comprehensive approach, including medication, dietary changes, weight management, regular exercise, and addressing underlying health conditions.

- **Individualized Care:** Each person's experience with gout is unique. Tailoring treatment plans to individual needs, taking into account age, gender, and overall health, is crucial for effective management and improved outcomes.

CHAPTER EIGHT

DEBUNKING COMMON MYTHS ABOUT GOUT AND DIE

Myth: All Proteins Are Bad for Gout

Fact: Not all proteins are created equal when it comes to gout. While high-purine proteins like red meat and seafood can trigger gout attacks, plant-based proteins and low-fat dairy products are generally considered safe. Moderation and a balanced approach to protein intake are key. Consult a healthcare provider or a dietitian for personalized dietary recommendations tailored to your specific needs.

Myth: Gout is Only Related to Diet

Fact: While diet plays a significant role in gout management, it's not the sole factor. Genetics, obesity, certain health conditions, and medications can also contribute. Managing gout effectively often requires a holistic approach, addressing lifestyle factors alongside dietary changes. Healthcare providers can provide comprehensive guidance on gout prevention and management.

Myth: Medication Alone Can Cure Gout

Fact: Medications are essential for managing gout symptoms and preventing attacks, but they are not a cure. Gout management also involves lifestyle changes, including dietary modifications, weight management, and regular exercise. Following a holistic treatment plan, as recommended by healthcare providers, is crucial for long-term gout control.

Myth: Gout is a Sign of Overindulgence

Fact: Gout is a medical condition influenced by various factors, including genetics and metabolism. While diet and lifestyle choices can contribute, gout is not solely a result of overindulgence. It can affect individuals with varying dietary habits and lifestyles. Understanding gout as a complex health issue helps reduce stigma and encourages supportive, empathetic approaches to its management.

CHAPTER NINE

RECIPES FOR A GOUT-FRIENDLY LIFESTYLE

Breakfast Ideas

1. Berry Yogurt Parfait:

Ingredients:

- 1 cup low-fat Greek yogurt
- 1/2 cup mixed berries (strawberries, blueberries, raspberries)
- 2 tablespoons honey or maple syrup (optional)
- 2 tablespoons granola (low-purine variety)

Instructions:

- In a glass or bowl, layer half of the yogurt.
- Add a layer of mixed berries on top of the yogurt.
- Drizzle with half of the honey or maple syrup (if using).
- Add the remaining yogurt as the next layer.
- Top with the rest of the berries, drizzle with the remaining honey or maple syrup, and sprinkle granola on top.
- Serve chilled.

Nutritional Information (approx.):

- Calories: 250-300
- Protein: 20g
- Carbohydrates: 40g
- Fiber: 6g
- Fat: 5g

2. Spinach and Mushroom Omelette:

Ingredients:

- 2 eggs, beaten
- 1/2 cup fresh spinach, chopped
- 1/4 cup mushrooms, sliced
- 1/4 cup low-fat cheese, grated
- Salt and pepper to taste
- 1 teaspoon olive oil

Instructions:

- Heat olive oil in a non-stick pan over medium heat.
- Add mushrooms and spinach, sauté until tender.
- Pour beaten eggs over the vegetables. Cook until the edges set.
- Sprinkle cheese, salt, and pepper over one half of the omelette.

- Fold the omelette in half and cook until the cheese melts.
- Serve hot.

Nutritional Information (approx.):

- Calories: 250-300
- Protein: 20g
- Carbohydrates: 4g
- Fiber: 1g
- Fat: 18g

3. Avocado Toast:

Ingredients:

- 1 slice whole-grain bread, toasted
- 1/2 ripe avocado, mashed
- Cherry tomatoes, sliced
- Sprinkle of chili flakes (optional)
- Fresh cilantro or parsley, chopped
- Salt and pepper to taste

Instructions:

- Spread mashed avocado evenly on the toasted bread.
- Top with sliced cherry tomatoes.
- Sprinkle with chili flakes (if using), fresh herbs, salt, and pepper.

- Serve immediately.

Nutritional Information (approx.):

- Calories: 200-250
- Protein: 5g
- Carbohydrates: 20g
- Fiber: 6g
- Fat: 15g

4. Greek Yogurt Smoothie:

Ingredients:

- 1 cup low-fat Greek yogurt
- 1/2 banana, frozen
- 1/2 cup mixed berries (strawberries, blueberries)
- 1 tablespoon chia seeds
- 1 teaspoon honey (optional)
- 1/2 cup water or unsweetened almond milk

Instructions:

- In a blender, combine Greek yogurt, frozen banana, mixed berries, chia seeds, honey (if using), and water/almond milk.
- Blend until smooth and creamy.
- Pour into a glass and serve immediately.

Nutritional Information (approx.):

- Calories: 250-300
- Protein: 20g
- Carbohydrates: 35g
- Fiber: 10g
- Fat: 7g

5. Quinoa Breakfast Bowl:

Ingredients:

- 1/2 cup cooked quinoa
- 1 tablespoon almond butter or peanut butter
- 1 tablespoon honey or maple syrup
- 1/2 banana, sliced
- 1 tablespoon chopped nuts (almonds, walnuts)
- Fresh berries for garnish

Instructions:

- In a bowl, combine cooked quinoa, almond butter, and honey/maple syrup. Mix well.
- Top with sliced banana, chopped nuts, and fresh berries.
- Drizzle with extra honey or maple syrup if desired.
- Serve warm or at room temperature.

Nutritional Information (approx.):

- Calories: 300-350

- Protein: 9g

- Carbohydrates: 50g

- Fiber: 6g

- Fat: 10g

Lunch Recipes

1. Grilled Chicken Salad:

Ingredients:

- 1 boneless, skinless chicken breast

- Mixed salad greens (spinach, arugula, lettuce)

- Cherry tomatoes, halved

- Cucumber, sliced

- Red onion, thinly sliced

- Olive oil and balsamic vinegar for dressing

- Salt and pepper to taste

Instructions:

- Season the chicken breast with salt and pepper, then grill until fully cooked.

- Slice the grilled chicken into strips.

- In a large bowl, combine the salad greens, cherry tomatoes, cucumber, and red onion.

- Drizzle with olive oil and balsamic vinegar, tossing gently to coat.

- Top the salad with grilled chicken strips.

- Serve immediately.

Nutritional Information (approx.):

- Calories: 300-350

- Protein: 30g

- Carbohydrates: 10g

- Fiber: 3g

- Fat: 15g

2. Quinoa and Vegetable Stir-Fry:

Ingredients:

- 1/2 cup cooked quinoa

- Mixed vegetables (bell peppers, broccoli, carrots), sliced

- Tofu or tempeh, cubed

- Low-sodium soy sauce

- Garlic powder and ginger powder for seasoning

- Green onions, chopped for garnish

Instructions:

- In a non-stick pan, stir-fry the tofu/tempeh until golden brown.
- Add the mixed vegetables and continue stir-frying until tender.
- Add cooked quinoa to the pan, season with garlic powder, and a splash of low-sodium soy sauce.
- Stir well until everything is heated through.
- Garnish with chopped green onions before serving.

Nutritional Information (approx.):

- Calories: 350-400
- Protein: 20g
- Carbohydrates: 40g
- Fiber: 7g
- Fat: 15g

3. Lentil Soup:

Ingredients:

- 1 cup dried lentils, rinsed and drained
- Onion, chopped
- Carrots, sliced
- Celery, chopped
- Low-sodium vegetable broth

- Garlic powder, cumin, and turmeric for seasoning
- Fresh parsley, chopped for garnish

Instructions:

- In a pot, sauté the chopped onion, carrots, and celery until softened.
- Add lentils and vegetable broth to the pot.
- Season with garlic powder, cumin, and turmeric. Bring to a boil.
- Reduce heat and simmer until lentils are tender and soup has thickened.
- Garnish with fresh parsley before serving.

Nutritional Information (approx.):

- Calories: 300-350
- Protein: 18g
- Carbohydrates: 55g
- Fiber: 16g
- Fat: 1g

4. Grilled Salmon with Quinoa and Steamed Vegetables:

Ingredients:

- 1 salmon fillet
- 1/2 cup cooked quinoa

- Mixed steamed vegetables (green beans, asparagus, zucchini)
- Lemon juice, olive oil, salt, and pepper for seasoning

Instructions:

- Season the salmon fillet with lemon juice, olive oil, salt, and pepper. Grill until cooked through.
- Serve the grilled salmon on a bed of cooked quinoa.
- Arrange steamed vegetables on the side.
- Drizzle with additional lemon juice and olive oil if desired.
- Serve hot.

Nutritional Information (approx.):

- Calories: 400-450
- Protein: 30g
- Carbohydrates: 30g
- Fiber: 6g
- Fat: 20g

5. Turkey and Avocado Wrap:

Ingredients:

- Whole-grain wrap or tortilla
- Sliced turkey breast

- Romaine lettuce leaves
- Avocado slices
- Tomato slices
- Low-fat Greek yogurt or hummus for spread
- Salt and pepper to taste

Instructions:

- Lay the whole-grain wrap on a clean surface.
- Spread a layer of Greek yogurt or hummus over the wrap.
- Arrange turkey slices, romaine lettuce, avocado slices, and tomato slices on top.
- Season with salt and pepper to taste.
- Roll the wrap tightly and cut in half diagonally.
- Serve immediately or wrap in parchment paper for a portable lunch.

Nutritional Information (approx.):

- Calories: 350-400
- Protein: 25g
- Carbohydrates: 40g
- Fiber: 8g
- Fat: 15g

Dinner Recipes

1. Baked Lemon Herb Chicken:

Ingredients:

- 2 boneless, skinless chicken breasts
- 1 lemon, juiced and zested
- 2 cloves garlic, minced
- 1 tablespoon fresh parsley, chopped
- 1 tablespoon olive oil
- Salt and pepper to taste

Instructions:

- Preheat the oven to 375°F (190°C).
- In a small bowl, mix lemon juice, lemon zest, minced garlic, chopped parsley, olive oil, salt, and pepper.
- Place chicken breasts in a baking dish and pour the lemon herb mixture over them.
- Bake for 25-30 minutes or until the chicken is cooked through.
- Serve hot with your choice of steamed vegetables or a green salad.

Nutritional Information (approx.):

- Calories: 250-300
- Protein: 30g

- Carbohydrates: 2g

- Fiber: 1g

- Fat: 14g

2. Shrimp and Vegetable Stir-Fry:

Ingredients:

- 1 pound shrimp, peeled and deveined

- Mixed vegetables (bell peppers, broccoli, snow peas), sliced

- 2 cloves garlic, minced

- 2 tablespoons low-sodium soy sauce

- 1 tablespoon sesame oil

- Green onions, chopped for garnish

- Sesame seeds for garnish

Instructions:

- Heat sesame oil in a pan or wok over medium-high heat.

- Add minced garlic and stir-fry until fragrant.

- Add shrimp and cook until they turn pink and opaque.

- Add mixed vegetables and stir-fry until they are tender yet crisp.

- Pour low-sodium soy sauce over the mixture and toss to combine.

- Garnish with chopped green onions and sesame seeds before serving.
- Serve hot over cooked brown rice or quinoa.

Nutritional Information (approx.):

- Calories: 300-350
- Protein: 25g
- Carbohydrates: 15g
- Fiber: 5g
- Fat: 15g

3. Grilled Vegetable and Tofu Skewers:

Ingredients:

- Firm tofu, cubed
- Mixed vegetables (bell peppers, zucchini, cherry tomatoes), cut into chunks
- 2 tablespoons olive oil
- 1 teaspoon cumin powder
- Salt and pepper to taste
- Fresh cilantro, chopped for garnish

Instructions:

- In a bowl, mix cubed tofu and mixed vegetables with olive oil, cumin powder, salt, and pepper.

- Thread tofu and vegetable chunks alternately onto skewers.
- Preheat the grill or grill pan over medium-high heat.
- Grill the skewers, turning occasionally, until the vegetables are tender and slightly charred.
- Garnish with fresh chopped cilantro before serving.
- Serve hot with a side of quinoa or a green salad.

Nutritional Information (approx.):

- Calories: 250-300
- Protein: 20g
- Carbohydrates: 15g
- Fiber: 5g
- Fat: 15g

4. Baked Salmon with Herb Crust:

Ingredients:

- 2 salmon fillets
- 1/4 cup fresh parsley, chopped
- 1/4 cup fresh dill, chopped
- 2 cloves garlic, minced
- 1 tablespoon olive oil
- Lemon zest from 1 lemon
- Salt and pepper to taste

Instructions:

- Preheat the oven to 400°F (200°C).
- In a bowl, combine chopped parsley, dill, minced garlic, olive oil, lemon zest, salt, and pepper.
- Place salmon fillets on a baking sheet lined with parchment paper.
- Press the herb mixture onto the top of each salmon fillet.
- Bake for 12-15 minutes or until the salmon is cooked through and flakes easily with a fork.
- Serve hot with a side of roasted vegetables or steamed asparagus.

Nutritional Information (approx.):

- Calories: 300-350
- Protein: 30g
- Carbohydrates: 2g
- Fiber: 1g
- Fat: 18g

5. Vegetable and Chickpea Curry:

Ingredients:

- 1 can chickpeas, drained and rinsed

- Mixed vegetables (bell peppers, cauliflower, peas), chopped
- 1 onion, finely chopped
- 2 cloves garlic, minced
- 1 can coconut milk
- 2 tablespoons curry powder
- 1 tablespoon olive oil
- Salt and pepper to taste
- Fresh cilantro, chopped for garnish

Instructions:

- Heat olive oil in a pot over medium heat. Add chopped onion and garlic, sauté until translucent.
- Add mixed vegetables and cook until slightly tender.
- Stir in chickpeas, curry powder, salt, and pepper.
- Pour in coconut milk and let the curry simmer for 15-20 minutes.
- Adjust seasoning as needed.
- Garnish with fresh chopped cilantro before serving.
- Serve hot over cooked brown rice or quinoa.

Nutritional Information (approx.):

- Calories: 300-350
- Protein: 10g

- Carbohydrates: 30g
- Fiber: 7g
- Fat: 20g

Snacks and Smoothies

1. Nutty Yogurt Parfait:

Ingredients:

- 1 cup low-fat Greek yogurt
- 2 tablespoons chopped almonds
- 2 tablespoons chopped walnuts
- 1 tablespoon honey or maple syrup
- Fresh berries for topping

Instructions:

- In a glass or bowl, layer half of the Greek yogurt.
- Sprinkle half of the chopped almonds and walnuts over the yogurt.
- Drizzle with half of the honey or maple syrup.
- Add the remaining yogurt as the next layer.
- Top with the rest of the nuts, drizzle with the remaining honey or maple syrup, and add fresh berries on top.
- Serve chilled.

Nutritional Information (approx.):

- Calories: 250-300
- Protein: 20g
- Carbohydrates: 20g
- Fiber: 3g
- Fat: 14g

2. Veggie Sticks with Hummus:

Ingredients

- Carrot sticks
- Celery sticks
- Cucumber slices
- Cherry tomatoes
- 1/2 cup hummus (low-fat variety)

Instructions:

- Wash and cut vegetables into sticks or slices.
- Serve the vegetable sticks with hummus for dipping.
- Enjoy this crunchy and satisfying snack.

Nutritional Information (approx.):

- Calories: 150-200
- Protein: 5g
- Carbohydrates: 20g

- Fiber: 6g

- Fat: 7g

3. Green Smoothie:

Ingredients:

- 1 cup spinach leaves

- 1/2 banana, frozen

- 1/2 cup pineapple chunks, frozen

- 1 tablespoon chia seeds

- 1 cup unsweetened almond milk

- 1 teaspoon honey (optional)

Instructions:

- In a blender, combine spinach, frozen banana, frozen pineapple chunks, chia seeds, almond milk, and honey (if using).

- Blend until smooth and creamy.

- Pour into a glass and serve immediately.

Nutritional Information (approx.):

- Calories: 200-250

- Protein: 6g

- Carbohydrates: 35g

- Fiber: 8g

- Fat: 7g

4. Cottage Cheese and Fruit Bowl:

Ingredients:

- 1/2 cup low-fat cottage cheese
- 1/2 cup mixed berries (strawberries, blueberries, raspberries)
- 1 tablespoon sliced almonds
- 1 teaspoon honey

Instructions:

- In a bowl, combine cottage cheese and mixed berries.
- Sprinkle sliced almonds on top and drizzle with honey.
- Mix gently and enjoy this protein-packed snack.

Nutritional Information (approx.):

- Calories: 200-250
- Protein: 20g
- Carbohydrates: 20g
- Fiber: 5g
- Fat: 8g

5. Berry Protein Smoothie:

Ingredients:

- 1/2 cup mixed berries (strawberries, blueberries, raspberries)

- 1 scoop low-purine protein powder
- 1 cup unsweetened almond milk
- 1 tablespoon flaxseeds
- 1 teaspoon honey (optional)

Instructions:

- In a blender, combine mixed berries, protein powder, almond milk, flaxseeds, and honey (if using).
- Blend until smooth and creamy.
- Pour into a glass and serve immediately.

Nutritional Information (approx.):

- Calories: 250-300
- Protein: 25g
- Carbohydrates: 20g
- Fiber: 6g
- Fat: 10g

Gout-Safe Desserts

1. Mixed Berry Yogurt Popsicles:

Ingredients:

- 1 cup mixed berries (strawberries, blueberries, raspberries)
- 1 cup low-fat Greek yogurt

- 2 tablespoons honey or maple syrup
- Popsicle molds and sticks

Instructions:

- In a blender, combine mixed berries, Greek yogurt, and honey/maple syrup. Blend until smooth.
- Pour the mixture into popsicle molds.
- Insert popsicle sticks and freeze for at least 4 hours or until solid.
- Remove from molds and enjoy these refreshing popsicles guilt-free.

Nutritional Information (approx. per popsicle):

- Calories: 80-100
- Protein: 5g
- Carbohydrates: 15g
- Fiber: 2g
- Fat: 1g

2. Baked Apples with Cinnamon:

Ingredients:

- 2 apples, cored and halved
- 1 tablespoon lemon juice
- 1 teaspoon ground cinnamon
- 1 tablespoon chopped nuts (almonds, walnuts)

- 1 tablespoon honey

Instructions:

- Preheat the oven to 375°F (190°C).
- Place apple halves in a baking dish, cut side up.
- Drizzle with lemon juice and sprinkle with cinnamon.
- Bake for 25-30 minutes or until apples are tender.
- Remove from the oven, sprinkle with chopped nuts, and drizzle with honey.
- Serve warm, optionally with a dollop of low-fat whipped cream.

Nutritional Information (approx. per serving):

- Calories: 150-180
- Protein: 2g
- Carbohydrates: 35g
- Fiber: 6g
- Fat: 3g

3. Chia Seed Pudding:

Ingredients:

- 3 tablespoons chia seeds
- 1 cup unsweetened almond milk
- 1 tablespoon honey or maple syrup

- Fresh berries for topping

Instructions:

- In a bowl, mix chia seeds, almond milk, and honey/maple syrup.
- Cover and refrigerate for at least 2 hours or overnight, allowing the chia seeds to absorb the liquid and form a pudding-like consistency.
- Stir well before serving.
- Top with fresh berries before serving.

Nutritional Information (approx. per serving):

- Calories: 150-180
- Protein: 4g
- Carbohydrates: 20g
- Fiber: 10g
- Fat: 7g

4. Banana-Oat Cookies:

Ingredients:

- 2 ripe bananas, mashed
- 1 cup old-fashioned oats
- 1/4 cup chopped nuts (pecans, almonds)
- 1/4 cup dark chocolate chips (optional)
- 1/2 teaspoon vanilla extract

- Pinch of salt

Instructions:

- Preheat the oven to 350°F (175°C).
- In a bowl, combine mashed bananas, oats, chopped nuts, chocolate chips (if using), vanilla extract, and a pinch of salt. Mix well.
- Drop spoonful of the mixture onto a baking sheet lined with parchment paper.
- Flatten each cookie slightly with the back of a fork.
- Bake for 12-15 minutes or until cookies are golden brown.
- Allow to cool before serving.

Nutritional Information (approx. per cookie):

- Calories: 80-100
- Protein: 2g
- Carbohydrates: 14g
- Fiber: 2g
- Fat: 3g

5. Frozen Banana Ice Cream:

Ingredients:

- 2 ripe bananas, peeled and sliced
- 1 tablespoon unsweetened cocoa powder

- 1/2 teaspoon vanilla extract
- 2 tablespoons chopped nuts (optional)

Instructions:

- Place banana slices in a freezer-safe container and freeze until solid, at least 2 hours.
- Transfer frozen banana slices to a blender or food processor.
- Add cocoa powder and vanilla extract. Blend until smooth and creamy, resembling the texture of ice cream.
- Serve immediately, topped with chopped nuts if desired.

Nutritional Information (approx. per serving):

- Calories: 100-120
- Protein: 2g
- Carbohydrates: 25g
- Fiber: 3g
- Fat: 1g

CONCLUSION

In conclusion, managing gout through dietary choices and a balanced lifestyle is not only achievable but also crucial for individuals seeking relief from this painful condition. Gout, caused by the buildup of uric acid crystals in the joints, can be effectively managed by understanding its underlying factors and implementing a gout-friendly diet and lifestyle.

We have explored various aspects of the gout diet, from understanding the condition itself to debunking common myths associated with gout. It's clear that gout is more than just a result of overindulgence; it's a complex interplay of genetics, lifestyle, and diet. Gout can affect people of all ages, genders, and backgrounds, and its management should be tailored to individual needs and circumstances.

The journey of gout management begins with education. Understanding what gout is, its causes, risk factors, symptoms, and potential complications is the first step toward better managing this condition. It's also crucial to dispel common misconceptions, such as the belief that all proteins are bad for gout. In fact, gout management requires a balanced approach to protein intake, among other dietary considerations.

Diet plays a significant role in gout management, with both foods to avoid and foods to include. Avoiding high-purine foods, red meat, and excessive alcohol can help reduce the risk of gout attacks. On the other hand, including anti-inflammatory foods, such as berries and leafy greens, can provide relief and reduce the frequency of flare-ups.

Balancing meals, weekly meal prep, portion control, and calorie management are key elements of an effective gout diet. Additionally, staying well-hydrated, increasing intake of Omega-3 fatty acids, and incorporating herbal teas can contribute to gout relief.

Lifestyle factors like regular exercise, stress management, and getting adequate sleep are equally important in gout management. Stress and poor sleep patterns can exacerbate gout symptoms, so implementing stress-reduction techniques and maintaining a healthy sleep routine can make a significant difference.

Lastly, regular medical checkups are essential to monitor gout progress and adjust treatment plans as needed.

We've also highlighted the unique considerations for different demographics, including gout in young adults, middle-aged individuals, seniors, and the specific challenges that women with gout may face.

In conclusion, a gout-friendly diet and lifestyle are powerful tools in managing gout effectively. With the right knowledge, dietary choices, and lifestyle adjustments, individuals can lead healthier, more comfortable lives while minimizing the impact of gout on their daily well-being.